Simplified Solution Approach

To PSORIASIS

Unlocking the Secrets to Clear, Radiant Skin: Your Comprehensive Guide to Lasting Relief and Renewal

Dr QUENTIN GLYN

Table Of Contents

CHAPTER ONE 6

Psoriasis 6

Definition: 6

Occurrence: 7

Effect On Life Quality: 8

CHAPTER TWO 12

Knowing About Psoriasis 12

Recognizing Psoriasis: 12

Reasons And Initiators: 13

Psoriasis Types: 14

Signs And Prognosis: 16

CHAPTER THREE 18

Traditional Interventions 18

1.   Topical Interventions: 18

2. Light Therapy, Or Phototherapy:...19

3. Medications For The System: 20

4. The Biologics: 21

5. Side Effects And Limitations: 22

CHAPTER FOUR 24

Lifestyle Modifications......................24

1.	Role Of Diet In Psoriasis:..........24

2. Techniques For Stress Management: 26

3. The Value Of Frequent Exercise: ..27

4. Effects Of Alcohol And Smoking: 28

CHAPTER FIVE 30

Home Treatments And Natural Remedies 30

1. Aloe Vera's Advantages:................30

2. Baths With Oatmeal:......................31

3. Psoriasis Essential Oils: 32

4. Supplements To The Diet: 33

5. Emollients And Moisturizers:........34

CHAPTER SIX......................36

Mind-Body Link 36

Mind-Body Link: 36

Psoriasis And Stress:......................37

Meditation & Mindfulness:................37

Methods Of Relaxation:....................39

Therapy Based On Cognitive Behavior (CBT):...39

Including The Mind-Body Method:...40

CHAPTER SEVEN 42

Holistic Methods For Treating Psoriasis42

1. Traditional Chinese Medicine (Tcm): 42

2. Ayurveda: 44

3. TCM:..46

4. Herbal Medicine: 47

CHAPTER EIGHT 50

Complementary Medicine 50

1. Blending Traditional And Non-Traditional Methods: 51

2. Team-Based Medical Care: 52

3. Treatment Plans Focused On The Patient: 54

CHAPTER NINE................................57

Individual Success Stories 57

Personal Success Tales: 57

Real-Life Experiences: 58

Testimonials:.......................................60

Lessons Learned: 61

Conclusion 63

Summary Of Crucial Techniques: 64

Providing Psoriasis Sufferers With
Empowerment:.....................................66

Considering The Future: 68

THE END 71

CHAPTER ONE

Psoriasis

Chronic autoimmune skin disease called psoriasis is characterized by a fast overproduction of skin cells that result in the development of thick, red, scaly patches. Millions of individuals worldwide suffer from this illness, which has a major negative influence on their quality of life. Although there isn't a cure for psoriasis, there are a number of treatment options that try to control symptoms and enhance a person's general quality of life.

Definition:

The inflammatory, non-contagious skin illness known as psoriasis is caused by an immune system dysfunction. T cells assist the immune system in defending the body against illness and infection. But with psoriasis, these T cells become hyperactive and set off an inflammatory reaction, which accelerates the proliferation of skin cells.

Occurrence:

People of all ages, colors, and genders are susceptible to psoriasis, which is a common ailment. Although the precise etiology of psoriasis is still unclear, environmental and genetic factors are important in its development. Global statistics indicate that 2-3% of people worldwide suffer with psoriasis. The frequency varies across various demographics and geographical areas.

Effect On Life Quality:

In addition to affecting the skin, psoriasis may have a significant negative effect on a person's general quality of life. Because psoriasis lesions are visible, they may cause humiliation, self-consciousness, and a diminished feeling of well-being. The following are some significant ways that psoriasis affects one's quality of life:

1. Effect on the body:

• Itching and pain: People with psoriasis may experience discomfort from itchy and painful lesions.

• Discomfort: The skin's redness and scaling may be physically uncomfortable and interfere with day-to-day activities.

2. Effect on the Mind:

• Stigma: Because psoriasis is visible, it may cause stigmatization, which lowers confidence and self-esteem.

• Emotional distress: Stress, anxiety, and depression may all be exacerbated by having a chronic skin problem.

3. Effect on Society:

• Social withdrawal: People with psoriasis may stop participating in social activities out of anxiety about their appearance and the stigma associated with it.

• Effect on relationships: Partners and family members may find it difficult to comprehend psoriasis, which may cause pressure in relationships.

4. Effect on Work:

• Difficulties at Work: People with psoriasis may encounter prejudice or difficulties at work as a result of misunderstandings regarding the ailment.

• Productivity: Psoriasis may have an adverse effect on job productivity and professional progress because of its physical and mental effects.

Comprehending the complex effects of psoriasis on people is essential to creating effective and comprehensive treatment strategies.

The quality of life for people with psoriasis may be greatly improved by a mix of medical therapies, lifestyle changes, and psychological support, while there isn't a single therapy that works for everyone.

To improve treatment choices for psoriasis sufferers and to better our knowledge of the condition, ongoing research and awareness campaigns are crucial.

CHAPTER TWO

Knowing About Psoriasis

Let's examine every facet of psoriasis knowledge, including kinds, symptoms, diagnosis, and causes and triggers.

Recognizing Psoriasis:

Psoriasis is a long-term autoimmune skin disorder that causes skin cells to divide more quickly. In psoriasis, skin cells renew themselves more quickly than they normally do—typically, every 10 to 30 days—which causes a buildup of cells on the skin's surface. Thick, scaly spots that may be red, itchy, and even painful are the result of this quick turnover.

Reasons And Initiators:

Genetics: Psoriasis has a significant hereditary component. The likelihood of having psoriasis rises if one or both parents have it.

Dysfunction of the Immune System: Because psoriasis is an autoimmune disease, healthy skin cells are wrongly attacked by the immune system. This results in inflammation and speeds up the growth of new skin cells.

Environmental variables: Psoriasis may be brought on by or made worse by certain environmental variables. These include skin injuries (such as cuts, burns, or bug bites), infections, and stress.

Medication: A number of medicines, including beta-blockers, lithium, and antimalarial treatments, may cause or exacerbate psoriasis.

Psoriasis Types:

Psoriasis plaque:

The most prevalent kind is described as having elevated, red areas that are coated in a silvery-white accumulation of dead skin cells.

Locations: Usually on the lower back, scalp, elbows, and knees.

Psoriasis with a guttate:

Small lesions resembling dots that are dispersed throughout the body.

Triggers: Bacterial illnesses such as streptococcal tonsillitis often cause them.

Psoriasis in reverse:

Red, smooth lesions appear in the folds of skin, such as the groin, armpits, and beneath the breasts.

Features: Generally less scaly than other varieties.

Psoriasis with pustules:

Blisters filled with pus and encircled by red skin.

Locations: Usually afflicted hands and feet.

Triggers: Medication side effects, systemic corticosteroid withdrawal, and infections may sometimes cause triggers.

Psoriasis erythrodermic:

Description: Skin that looks like it has been severely burned, with widespread redness and scaling.

Severity: Because of the possibility of systemic consequences, it is regarded as a medical emergency.

Signs And Prognosis:

Signs:

Skin that is crimson in places and coated with thick, silvery scales.

Chapped, dry skin that might bleed.

Soreness, burning, or itching.

Pitted or thickened nails.

Stiff and swollen joints (perhaps psoriatic arthritis).

Conclusion:

Often determined by looking at the patient's medical history and skin.

A skin biopsy might be done to verify the diagnosis.

There is no particular blood test for psoriasis, however, other illnesses may be ruled out using testing.

To sum up, psoriasis is a complicated disease with a wide range of forms and causes. It is essential to comprehend these elements in order to manage the illness and create successful treatment strategies.

CHAPTER THREE
Traditional Interventions

Let's explore the standard therapies for psoriasis and the simpler solution method. Psoriasis is a long-term autoimmune skin disease that causes red, scaly areas due to a fast accumulation of skin cells. Traditional therapies include a variety of approaches, each focusing on certain facets of the illness.

1. Topical Interventions:

• Corticosteroids: For mild to moderate psoriasis, these anti-inflammatory medications are frequently prescribed. In the afflicted regions, they function by lowering inflammation and inhibiting the immunological response.

• Topical Retinoids: Made from vitamin A, retinoids reduce inflammation and slow down the growth of new skin cells. To increase their efficacy, they are often combined with other therapies.

• Calcineurin Inhibitors: Topical immunosuppressive drugs such as tacrolimus and pimecrolimus are especially helpful in delicate areas such as the face and genitalia.

2. Light Therapy, Or Phototherapy:

• UVB Phototherapy: UVB light exposure helps reduce the uncontrollably high rate of skin cell growth. It can be taken either on its own or in conjunction with other treatments, and it is administered in a controlled setting.

• PUVA Therapy: Another type of phototherapy uses psoralen in conjunction with UVA light. Psoralen, which helps to slow down skin cell growth, is applied topically or taken internally by patients prior to exposure to UVA light.

3. Medications For The System:

• Methotrexate: For severe psoriasis, this immunosuppressive drug is frequently prescribed. It functions by stifling the immune system and preventing the skin cells from growing rapidly.

• Cyclosporine: Because of its possible adverse effects, cyclosporine is usually only used temporarily. It is an immunosuppressant that lowers the immune response and is useful for treating severe psoriasis.

4. The Biologics:

• TNF Inhibitors: To lessen inflammation, tumor necrosis factor (TNF) inhibitors, including adalimumab and etanercept, target certain immune system proteins. They are usually saved for moderate to severe cases and are provided via injection.

• Inhibitors of IL-17 and IL-23: These more recent biologics, such as ixekizumab and secukinumab, target certain proteins implicated in the inflammatory process of psoriasis, providing tailored treatment with fewer adverse effects.

5. Side Effects And Limitations:

• Topical Treatments: Side effects may include skin thinning (with corticosteroids), irritation, and mild burning. Long-term usage might develop resistance.

• Phototherapy: Potential adverse effects include sunburn, accelerated aging, and an increased risk of skin cancer with long-term usage.

• Systemic Medications: Methotrexate and cyclosporine may have serious adverse effects, including liver and kidney damage, and an increased risk of infection.

• Biologics: While typically well-tolerated, biologics may raise the risk of infections and have related expenses.

In conclusion, the choice of therapy relies on the severity of psoriasis, personal preferences, and probable side effects. A tailored strategy, sometimes incorporating a mix of medications, is usual for efficiently controlling psoriasis while reducing side effects and restrictions. Regular monitoring and contact with healthcare experts are necessary for effective long-term treatment.

CHAPTER FOUR
Lifestyle Modifications

Psoriasis is a chronic autoimmune illness marked by the fast accumulation of skin cells, resulting in red, scaly areas. While medical treatments play a key role, lifestyle adjustments may considerably help to treat psoriasis symptoms and increase general well-being.

1. Role Of Diet In Psoriasis:

Anti-Inflammatory Foods: Incorporating an anti-inflammatory diet may help minimize psoriasis symptoms. Pay attention to foods high in omega-3 fatty acids, such as walnuts, flaxseeds, and fatty fish (like mackerel and salmon).

Brightly Colored Fruits and Veggies: Consuming a lot of fruits and veggies gives you important antioxidants, vitamins, and minerals. These nutrients have the ability to lower inflammation and improve skin health.

Reducing Food Triggers: Some people may discover that certain foods make their psoriasis symptoms worse. Dairy, gluten, and red meat are common causes. Recognizing and avoiding certain stressors may be advantageous.

Hydration: Maintaining enough hydration is crucial for healthy skin. Water may relieve psoriasis-related dryness and preserve the suppleness of the skin.

2. Techniques For Stress Management:

Meditation and mindfulness: These techniques help lower stress levels, which may lessen the symptoms of psoriasis. Mind-body practices, such as tai chi and yoga, may also be helpful.

Exercises for Deep Breathing: By triggering the body's relaxation response, deep breathing techniques assist in lowering stress. Including methods like diaphragmatic breathing may be quite beneficial.

Time management: Overwhelming stress may be avoided by effectively managing time and establishing reasonable objectives.

This entails setting priorities for your work and taking pauses when required.

therapy and Support Groups: Joining a support group or obtaining professional therapy may provide coping mechanisms and emotional support to help manage the difficulties of having psoriasis.

3. The Value Of Frequent Exercise:

Cardiovascular Exercise: Walking, running, and swimming are examples of cardiovascular exercises that enhance blood circulation, which is essential for healthy skin. A healthy weight may be maintained with exercise as well.

Strength Training: Increasing muscular mass with strength training may improve general health and strengthen the immune system.

Joint Flexibility: Psoriatic arthritis, a kind of joint discomfort, has been linked to psoriasis. Frequent exercise that incorporates flexibility training and stretches may enhance joint function and lessen stiffness.

4. Effects Of Alcohol And Smoking:

Smoking: Research has shown that smoking aggravates pre-existing psoriasis symptoms and increases the chance of getting the condition. Reducing smoking may have a major positive impact on the severity of psoriasis and the effectiveness of therapy.

Alcohol Use: Consuming too much alcohol may reduce the efficacy of certain drugs and is linked to an increased risk of psoriasis. Alcohol use for psoriasis sufferers may need to be moderated or avoided completely.

In summary, a comprehensive strategy that incorporates lifestyle changes may enhance medicinal interventions and improve the management of psoriasis. Psoriasis sufferers must collaborate closely with medical specialists to create a customized strategy that takes into account their particular requirements and situation.

CHAPTER FIVE

Home Treatments And Natural Remedies

Psoriasis is a long-term skin disorder characterized by red, scaly, and itchy skin patches. Even while there are medicinal options, a lot of people go for over-the-counter and natural solutions to control their symptoms and maintain healthy skin. Here's a thorough rundown of some of the main ideas behind this strategy:

1. Aloe Vera's Advantages:

Anti-Inflammatory Characteristics: Aloe vera has long been recognized for its ability to decrease inflammation and redness brought on by psoriasis.

Moisturizing Effect: Aloe vera gel soothes dry, irritated skin by acting as a cooling and moisturizing agent.

Application: Use skincare products containing aloe vera or simply apply pure aloe vera gel to the afflicted areas.

2. Baths With Oatmeal:

Calming Qualities: Oatmeal is well known for having anti-inflammatory and calming qualities on the skin. It may lessen inflammation and ease itching.

To prepare, add colloidal oatmeal to a warm bath and let it soak for fifteen to twenty minutes. Regular use of this may help control psoriasis symptoms.

Pat Dry: To prevent irritation, gently pat the skin dry after taking an oatmeal bath.

3. Psoriasis Essential Oils:

Tea Tree Oil: Well-known for its anti-inflammatory and antifungal qualities, tea tree oil may help reduce the symptoms of psoriasis. Before using, dilute it to prevent irritation.

Lavender Oil: Having calming properties, lavender oil may help lower stress levels, which may lead to flare-ups of psoriasis.

Application: Apply a combination of essential oils and carrier oils, such as jojoba or coconut, to the regions that are impacted.

Before implementing widely, do a patch test.

4. Supplements To The Diet:

Omega-3 Fatty Acids: Rich in flaxseed oil, walnuts, and fish oil, omega-3 fatty acids contain anti-inflammatory qualities that may help those who suffer from psoriasis.

Vitamin D: Because this vitamin is important for healthy skin, some research indicates that taking supplements may help control the symptoms of psoriasis.

Consultation: Prior to adding new supplements to your regimen, always get advice from a medical practitioner.

5. Emollients And Moisturizers:

Moisture: Maintaining healthy moisture levels in the skin is essential for controlling psoriasis.

Flare-ups and worsening symptoms might be caused by dry skin.

Selecting Products: Look for emollients and moisturizers that are hypoallergenic and devoid of smell. After taking a bath, use these to seal in moisture.

Components to look for: To encourage skin hydration, look for components in moisturizers including ceramides, hyaluronic acid, and shea butter.

Although home therapies and natural cures might be helpful in treating the symptoms of psoriasis, it's important to keep in mind that each person's reaction may be different. A dermatologist or other medical expert should be consulted before beginning any new treatment plan.

For a more all-encompassing approach to psoriasis care, these natural methods may be enhanced by leading a healthy lifestyle, controlling stress, and avoiding irritants.

CHAPTER SIX
Mind-Body Link

In order to effectively manage and cure psoriasis, the mind-body link is essential. Psoriasis is a chronic skin illness that is impacted by a number of variables. Developing a simpler solution approach may be made easier by having a better grasp of how the mind and body interact.

Mind-Body Link:

The complex interrelationship between mental and physical health is highlighted by the mind-body link. The intensity and worsening of psoriasis symptoms have been shown to be significantly influenced by stress and emotional well-being. In order to address the mind-body link, psychological elements that may be involved in the onset and course of psoriasis must be identified and managed.

Psoriasis And Stress:

Stress is a major cause of flare-ups in psoriasis. Stress may modify the immune system's reaction in people, which may exacerbate psoriasis symptoms and cause inflammation. Therefore, a significant element of a streamlined treatment approach to psoriasis is stress management.

Meditation & Mindfulness:

Techniques for mindfulness and meditation are useful strategies for reducing stress.

While meditation encourages calmness and mental clarity, mindfulness focuses on being in the present moment without passing judgment. People with psoriasis may be able to better control their stress levels and maybe lessen the frequency and intensity of flare-ups by incorporating mindfulness techniques into their everyday lives.

Deep breathing exercises, guided meditation, and careful awareness of one's thoughts and emotions are a few examples of mindfulness practices. These methods provide a positive outlook, which is advantageous for general well-being, in addition to helping to reduce stress.

Methods Of Relaxation:

To reduce tension and foster calm, a variety of relaxation methods may be used. A psoriasis treatment strategy might include relaxation methods such as progressive muscle relaxation, deep breathing exercises, and visualization. By inducing the body's relaxation response, these methods seek to offset the physiological impacts of stress and support a more balanced immune system.

Therapy Based On Cognitive Behavior (CBT):

A treatment strategy called cognitive behavioral therapy aims to recognize and change harmful thinking patterns and behaviors. When it comes to psoriasis, cognitive behavioral therapy (CBT) may assist patients in stress management, emotional coping, and the development of healthy thought patterns. CBT may enhance psychological well-being by addressing maladaptive beliefs and behaviors, which may have a beneficial effect on psoriasis symptoms.

Including The Mind-Body Method:

A comprehensive strategy for managing psoriasis entails incorporating the mind-body link into daily living. Combining mindfulness exercises, stress management strategies, and therapeutic therapies like cognitive behavioral therapy (CBT) may be part of this. It's vital to remember that different people may find these strategies to be more or less successful, so creating a customized strategy that takes into account each person's particular requirements and preferences is essential.

In conclusion, a simple solution approach to psoriasis must acknowledge and treat the mind-body relationship. People may improve their mental and physical health by practicing stress management, mindfulness and relaxation methods, and cognitive behavioral tactics. This can result in a more thorough and successful psoriasis treatment strategy.

CHAPTER SEVEN

Holistic Methods For Treating Psoriasis

Psoriasis is a long-term autoimmune disease that causes red, scaly patches to appear on the skin and inflammation. While topical steroids, phototherapy, and systemic drugs are often offered as traditional medical therapies for psoriasis, some people prefer holistic and alternative methods. We'll discuss holistic methods here, such as acupuncture, herbal medicine, Ayurveda, and Traditional Chinese Medicine (TCM).

1. Traditional Chinese Medicine (Tcm):

The foundation of TCM is the

notion that Qi, or life force, and the opposing energies of Yin and Yang must be in balance for one to be healthy. According to TCM, psoriasis is an indication of a bodily imbalance. The goals of TCM treatments are to promote general health and bring this equilibrium back. Important elements of TCM for psoriasis consist of:

• Acupuncture: According to Traditional Chinese Medicine, acupuncture stimulates energy flow and restores balance by placing tiny needles into certain body locations. According to some research, acupuncture may be able to lessen the severity of psoriasis lesions and aid with symptoms.

• Herbal Medicine: Chinese herbal medicines often include combining different herbs according to each person's unique symptoms and constitution. Teas, powders, or tablets may be used to deliver these. Clinical research has shown that some plants, such as Indigo naturalis, may be promising in treating psoriasis.

• Dietary Adjustments: To treat the underlying imbalances causing psoriasis, Traditional Chinese Medicine (TCM) practitioners may suggest certain dietary adjustments. This may include eating meals that support balance and avoiding items thought to aggravate inflammation.

2. Ayurveda: According to this age-old Indian medical system, vata, pitta, and kapha doshas should be in balance for optimal health. According to Ayurveda, psoriasis is often linked to a Pitta dosha imbalance. Among the ayurvedic treatments for psoriasis are:

• Food and Lifestyle Adjustments: Ayurveda places a strong emphasis on food adjustments according to a person's dosha constitution. Eat less of the foods that irritate Pitta, such as spicy and acidic meals. Additionally, stress is modifications to one's lifestyle, such as frequent exercise and stress reduction.

• Herbal Remedies: Due to their anti-inflammatory and skin-soothing qualities, Ayurvedic herbs like neem, turmeric, and aloe vera are often utilized. It could be advised to use herbal supplements, oils, or pastes.

• Panchakarma: In Ayurveda, this cleansing procedure tries to get rid of toxins from the body. Panchakarma treatments might include cleaning techniques, herbal steam treatments, and massage.

3. TCM: TCM includes acupuncture, which is the insertion of tiny needles into certain body sites. In relation to psoriasis:

• Regulating Qi Flow: It is thought that acupuncture might help balance out Qi imbalances that may be causing symptoms of psoriasis. It could potentially have effects on immunomodulation.

• Stress Reduction: It is well recognized that stress and relaxation are elements that contribute to flare-ups of psoriasis.

Acupuncture treatments may help with these goals.

4. Herbal Medicine: In both TCM and Ayurveda, herbal medicine is an important part of holistic psoriasis treatment.

• Anti-Inflammatory Herbs: Due to their well-known anti-inflammatory qualities, herbs including licorice, aloe vera, chamomile, and turmeric may be able to reduce the symptoms of psoriasis.

• Herbs that Modulate the Immune System: Certain herbs, including reishi mushrooms and astragalus in Traditional Chinese Medicine, are thought to modify the immune system, which may help with the autoimmune component of psoriasis that underlies it.

• Topical Herbal Applications: To relieve skin irritation and lessen inflammation, use lotions or ointments containing herbal extracts topically.

It's crucial to remember that although holistic methods help a lot of individuals, everyone reacts differently. It is best to speak with medical specialists before using these methods, particularly if you are already receiving traditional therapy for psoriasis. Integrative therapy, which blends traditional and holistic methods, could provide a thorough approach to psoriasis management.

CHAPTER EIGHT

Complementary Medicine

Psoriasis is a long-term autoimmune disease that causes red, scaly spots on the skin due to a fast accumulation of skin cells. Psoriasis management often calls for an all-encompassing strategy.

By integrating traditional and alternative methods, encouraging team-based care, and customizing treatment regimens for each patient, integrative medicine emerges as a viable answer.

1. Blending Traditional And Non-Traditional Methods:

The focus of integrative medicine is on how complementary therapies and traditional medical care may work together. Conventional therapies aim to reduce symptoms by targeting the immune system, such as systemic medicines, phototherapy, and topical corticosteroids. However, by treating underlying causes of psoriasis-like inflammation and stress, complementary therapies including acupuncture, dietary changes, and herbal supplements may enhance traditional therapy.

•	Conventional Therapies: Topical medications such as corticosteroids or vitamin D analogs are often prescribed by dermatologists. Systemic drugs such as immunosuppressants or biologics may be advised in more severe situations.

•	Alternative Therapies: Dietary modifications, meditation, and acupuncture may all help reduce inflammation and stress. Natural treatments such as fish oil supplements or aloe vera help some individuals feel better.

2. Team-Based Medical Care:

A multidisciplinary team approach combining dermatologists, primary care doctors, nurses, mental health specialists, and practitioners of alternative medicine is beneficial for the therapy of psoriasis. Every team member has a distinct area of expertise to handle various facets of the illness and how it affects the patients' general health.

• Dermatologists: Offer proficiency in standard care, tracking the progress of illnesses, and modifying drug schedules.

• Primary treatment Physicians: Are essential in managing comorbidities, coordinating treatment with other specialists, and overseeing overall health care.

• Mental Health Professionals: Provide assistance for coping mechanisms and stress reduction in order to help manage the psychological effects of psoriasis.

• Practitioners of Alternative Medicine: Offer comprehensive viewpoints, combining treatments such as naturopathy or acupuncture to improve general health.

3. Treatment Plans Focused On The Patient:

Integrative medicine's core tenet is treating patients as individuals with unique needs. Since every individual is affected by psoriasis differently, patient-centered treatment entails active cooperation between medical professionals and patients to create customized plans that fit objectives, preferences, and lifestyles.

• Individualized Assessments: When creating treatment regimens, medical professionals take into account the patient's preferences, the severity of their psoriasis, and the existence of any comorbidities.

• Shared Decision-Making: Patients who are well-informed are able to actively engage in treatment choices, ensuring that the therapies they choose are consistent with their beliefs and way of life.

• Lifestyle Adjustments: Integrative medicine encourages patients to take up stress-reduction techniques, consistent exercise regimens, and dietary adjustments, all of which may help reduce the symptoms of psoriasis.

Through the smooth integration of traditional and alternative medicines, the promotion of team-based care, and the prioritization of patient-centered treatment regimens, integrative medicine offers a simpler solution approach to psoriasis. This all-encompassing approach improves the entire quality of life for those who suffer from psoriasis by addressing not just the physical symptoms but also the psychological and emotional ones.

CHAPTER NINE
Individual Success Stories

For those with psoriasis, using success stories, firsthand accounts, endorsements, and life lessons may provide insightful information and motivation. Let's examine each idea in more detail:

Personal Success Tales: People who are going through comparable difficulties may get great inspiration and motivation from personal success tales. People who have effectively controlled their psoriasis may talk about their experiences, going into depth about the highs and lows, tactics they used, and achievements they made. Success stories may demonstrate the range of experiences and the fact that there isn't a single psoriasis treatment that works for everyone. Among the crucial components these tales should include are:

Early difficulties and hardships.

Moments of awareness or turning points.

The procedure for looking for and locating efficient therapies.

Alterations in lifestyle that helped things become better.

Successes and successes in spite of having psoriasis.

Real-Life Experiences: Psoriasis patients' daily struggles and victories are shown when they share their real-life experiences. This might include talking about the ways that psoriasis impacts relationships, jobs, social life, and everyday activities. Individuals may better empathize with others' problems and comprehend the practical elements of treating psoriasis by drawing on their own experiences. Some subjects to look into are:

Coping strategies for mental and physical difficulties.

Techniques for managing tension and episodes.

Navigating social circumstances and getting beyond stigma.

Juggling other obligations in life with self-care.

assembling a network of friends, family, and medical experts for support.

Testimonials: Testimonials provide people a way to voice their happiness with certain medical interventions, way-of-life adjustments, or healthcare practitioners. They may provide hope to others who are still looking for answers and act as proof of the efficacy of certain strategies. When writing testimonials, think about incorporating:

Specifics of the successful course of action or therapy.

The treatment's effects on both mental and physical health.

Alterations in life quality after the use of a certain tactic.

Suggestions for others with comparable difficulties.

Recognition of the important role that healthcare workers perform.

Lessons Learned: Those who manage their psoriasis may benefit much from the knowledge gained from this experience. These lessons may be applied to both achievements and failures, and they can be very helpful in pointing people in the direction of more sensible management techniques. Some things to think about learning may be:

The value of patient advocacy in the medical field.

Being tenacious and patient in finding the best course of action.

Adopting a holistic perspective on health, this includes mental wellness.

Identifying triggers and selecting a lifestyle that suits oneself.

The importance of creating a solid support network.

A thorough and approachable resource may be made by combining testimonies, real-life experiences, success stories, and lessons gained. This collection may provide a multifaceted viewpoint on psoriasis management and life, encouraging a feeling of empowerment and camaraderie among those dealing with comparable issues.

Conclusion

To sum up, treating psoriasis with a simple solution requires a multimodal approach that includes both medical treatments and all-encompassing care for those who have the condition. In addition to treating the physical symptoms, empowering those who suffer from psoriasis and encouraging a proactive mentality are crucial steps in controlling and lessening the condition's effects. As we go through the complications of psoriasis, it becomes clear that improving the quality of life for people who have the condition over the long term requires a holistic strategy.

Summary Of Crucial Techniques:

1. Medical Procedures:

• Seek prompt medical diagnosis and guidance.

• Work together with medical experts to investigate appropriate therapy choices, such as topical remedies, systemic drugs, and biologics.

• Regularly assessing symptoms and modifying treatment regimens as necessary.

• Include lifestyle adjustments including stress management, avoiding triggers, and eating a balanced diet.

2. Comprehensive Methods:

• To improve general well-being, embrace alternative treatments like phototherapy, acupuncture, or meditation.

• Create a supportive atmosphere by teaching friends and family about psoriasis and how to manage it.

• Promote mental health services, such as therapy or support groups, to help with the emotional side of having a chronic illness.

3. Self-Management and Lifestyle Adjustments:

• Create and follow a skincare regimen to control psoriatic lesions.

• Make stress reduction a top priority by engaging in exercises, yoga, and mindfulness practices.

• Eat a healthy, well-balanced diet to promote the health of your skin.

Providing Psoriasis Sufferers With Empowerment:

An essential component of psoriasis management is empowerment. This entails giving patients the information, abilities, and self-assurance they need to take an active role in their care and everyday activities. Among the empowerment techniques are:

1. Learning:

• Assure people have access to correct information on psoriasis, including its causes and treatments.

• Encourage awareness of triggers and practical management techniques.

2. Self-Observation:

• Motivate people to monitor their symptoms and response to therapy.

• Encourage honest dialogue with medical professionals so that treatment plans may be modified on time.

3. Lobbying:

• Assist people in voicing their concerns to the healthcare system.

• Promote participation in patient advocacy organizations to spread knowledge and influence legislative decisions.

Considering The Future:

With further developments in medical research, technology, and an increasing focus on holistic well-being, the treatment of psoriasis has a bright future. Important things to think about in the future are:

1. Novel Therapies:

• Ongoing investigation into cutting-edge therapeutics, such as gene-based and customized medicine.

• Investigating cutting-edge technology, including telemedicine, to increase access to medical services.

2. Improved Assistance for Patients:

• Creation of specialized support plans that cater to the particular requirements of psoriasis sufferers.

• Using digital health technology to provide individualized treatment plans and remote monitoring.

3. Taking Stigma Down:

• Promotion of greater knowledge and comprehension of psoriasis in order to lessen social stigma.

• Fostering acceptance and inclusiveness for those with visible skin problems.

Simplifying the treatment of psoriasis essentially necessitates a dynamic blend of empowerment tactics, holistic support, and medical developments.

In order to reduce the effects of psoriasis and enable those who are afflicted to lead satisfying lives, we must actively engage people in their treatment and promote a thorough awareness of the condition.

THE END